Getting Ready for Birth

A Short and Empowering Guide to Labor in Any Setting

Maris Young
Young Creative Enterprises

Getting Ready for Birth: A Short and Empowering Guide to Labor in Any Setting
ISBN: 979-8-9988522-2-0

First Edition
Cover design by: Maris Young
Interior design by: Maris Young

Published by: Young Creative Enterprises

For permissions, inquiries or to connect with the author, please visit: youngcreativeenterprises.com

Dedication

To the ones preparing to give birth. To the ones who already have. To those who feel they have forgotten, and to those who are learning to remember.

May this book be a compass back to honoring the sacred and transformative power of giving birth.

Table of Contents

Introduction

My name is Maris Young, and I'm a wife, mother, breastfeeding consultant, childbirth educator and a certified doula who supports families through pre-conception, pregnancy, birth and postpartum. As a doula, I share evidence-based information to help my clients make informed decisions about their care. I share reassuring encouragement, teach holistic relaxation modalities, hold a safe space to be heard and provide a calm, non-judgmental presence throughout the fertility journey. And I also share loving touch and hands-on comfort techniques while providing continuous support whether my clients choose to birth at home, at a birth center or at the hospital.

I wrote this book as a short and simple guide to help you navigate labor in any setting. First, a little about me.

Becoming a mother in 2017 catapulted me into an existential crisis. And all of a sudden, I felt a deep need to make sense of the physical, mental, emotional and spiritual shifts I had experienced from pregnancy through early postpartum. So, I began to study. The more I learned, the more I realized that this wisdom is truly our birthright as humans. Yet, when I looked around, so many people were in the dark about the sacred act of childbearing. I vowed to hold the torch for honest conversations to follow, and Young Honest Mother was born, manifesting first as a personal blog and then as a podcast.

I produced Young Honest Mother: The Podcast from July 2019 until December 2020 fueled by a passion to protect others from feeling monumentally unprepared for the reality of marriage, motherhood and modern home economics. I invited industry experts and everyday women onto the show to share their stories and the gems they mined from them. Most of the conversations I featured on the podcast were with people I had never spoken to before: single mothers, former teen mothers, divorced mothers, widows, wives, doctors, doulas.

The birth of my second child in 2022 introduced me to a local nonprofit aiming to improve the unfortunate maternal outcomes in my community. In 2023, I completed doula training that highlighted providing trauma-informed care that is also compassionate and culturally respectful. In 2024, that same local nonprofit contracted me to offer free doula services to a largely under-resourced population in the zip code with the second highest maternal mortality rate in my state. I also happened to be pregnant with my third child during my first official year of serving as a doula and while writing this book. So, I had the unique opportunity to help others get ready for birth while getting ready for birth myself.

As a doula, I guide my clients through pregnancy, translate medical jargon, hold space for big emotions, troubleshoot breastfeeding issues, advocate for my clients' wishes and more. I also offer loving on-site support during births in a variety of different scenarios ranging from scheduled c-sections, unplanned c-sections, emergency c-sections and both unmedicated and medicated vaginal births at hospitals, birth centers and at clients' homes. In seeing great need for my clients to be connected with community resources from pregnancy to parenthood, I co-created Maternal Resource Oasis to bridge the gap.

This book is inspired by my own three beautiful births and my work as a doula. When I'm working with doula clients, I lead them through a series of consultations designed to educate them on the foundational elements of getting ready for birth. After each hour-long session, many of my clients tell me how grateful they were to have learned so much and how they wished they could have packaged up everything I was teaching so that they could go back and review it later. This book, *Getting Ready for Birth*, is my way of doing just that.

Too many women have found themselves unprepared for the sacred act of childbearing, leaving themselves at the mercy of a medical system that at times prioritizes protocols and profits over compassion. I am offering a different narrative, one where women move toward birth feeling more at ease because they are empowered with the insights to make informed decisions about their prenatal care.

This book is for those who are getting ready for birth of any kind (vaginal, medicated, c-section, home birth, birth center or hospital) and for those who know someone who is. I recommend using this book as a companion guide to reference alongside working with your own doula. A doula will be able to offer personalized support, and they can help you put the information in this book into practice for your unique childbearing circumstances.

My goal is that by the end of this book, you'll know how to:
- classify the stages of labor in order to better visualize what your body could experience while bringing new life into the world.
- train your mind for birth in order to improve mental endurance.
- create your own Birth Vision in order to gain clarity about your birthing preferences.
- explore different birth possibilities in order to be prepared with vital insights in case your birthing experience isn't quite what you envisioned.

Let's begin!

Chapter 1: Shift Your Perception of Labor

To start, it's important to be aware of how you view labor and birth. Many of my clients have told me that they're afraid of what labor will feel like because they've heard so many accounts of miserably painful birth experiences. This perspective on birth has even been reinforced by movies and TV shows. In all honesty, labor can be enjoyable and even orgasmic. I've experienced it myself. (But that's a topic for another book!) It starts by making the shift to transform the way you perceive your experience.

You can choose how you perceive and respond to the sensations in your body, even during birth. The way you perceive the contractions influences the way you respond to them. And since you can choose how you perceive your experience, I encourage you to connect the idea of labor with more positive feelings. Here's how.

For example, a laboring mother who perceives contractions as "painful" might feel like doing whatever she can to avoid experiencing those sensations. Keep in mind that when we're fighting against something, when we're fearful, our bodies tense up. That's the exact opposite of what we want to happen when we're giving birth. Instead, we want our bodies to open. And when you are moving into labor with the energy of "No! I don't like this! Make it stop!" you're speaking against what needs to happen in order for you to birth your baby. And that tension also makes it more challenging for your cervix to dilate.

On the other hand, a laboring mother who perceives contractions as "helpful" might approach the labor sensations with a sense of gratitude and acceptance. When I gave birth to my second child, I welcomed the contractions and softened into the labor sensations which allowed my cervix to dilate more effectively. I went into labor with the energy of "Yes! This is exactly what I need! Open!" which helped me to remember that the contractions were there to help me meet my baby.

When you commit to making this conscious shift in perception, you can transform the way you perceive your experience. It is, indeed, possible to experience birth as enjoyable and even orgasmic.

Chapter 2: Learning Labor

Most of my clients expected that they would learn the ins and outs of labor from their doctors. Those very same clients were shocked to realize that there wasn't time to learn much of anything during their short prenatal appointments. As a childbirth educator, I have witnessed how learning about labor helps my clients to feel more comfortable and at ease as they're getting ready for birth, whether it is their first baby or not.

In fact, I had the honor of supporting a client during the pregnancy of her 8th child. I asked her to let me know if any of this information was redundant because I didn't want to waste her time. I was surprised when she told me that she had never learned any of the labor signs during her previous pregnancies! Learning the foundational elements of what labor is all about helps women to get ready for birth, increasing their confidence about what the experience can look and feel like.

So, by the end of this section, you'll be able to:
- identify different signs that you're going into labor.
- categorize the labor stages.
- recognize when it's time to go to your birthing location.
- choose techniques that can help you feel more comfortable during labor.

Labor Signs
Losing the Mucus Plug
I like to think of the mucus plug like the cork in a wine bottle. During pregnancy, the mucus plug seals off the cervix to keep bacteria from entering the uterus and causing an infection, much like a cork keeps things from getting into the wine bottle. As you get closer to the baby being born, the cervix begins to thin (efface) and open (dilate). Eventually, there won't be enough pressure to hold the mucus plug in place. So, losing the mucus plug is a sign that your cervix is changing and getting ready for birth.

When birth is near, you'll start to notice the mucus plug coming out after you wipe. It looks very much like the kind of mucus you might see when you're blowing your nose, greenish yellow with tinges of pink or red on the edges. This jelly-like glob can be expelled all at once or little by little over a few days' time. Labor contractions tend to start soon after the mucus plug is expelled.

Water Breaking

When the amniotic sac that surrounds the baby ruptures, we say that someone's water is breaking. Most people have seen women going into labor on TV shows or movies. To make the experience more dramatic and screen-worthy, there's usually a big moment where the pregnant woman's water breaks. This is how a lot of people come to associate the water breaking with going into labor. In reality, you can be in labor even if your water hasn't broken!

For some women, the water breaks, and then labor contractions begin immediately. Sometimes the rupture is big and dramatic and other times women experience a slow leaking of amniotic fluid that continues over a period of days. Other women may have labor contractions and be close to fully dilated before their water breaks. And in rare cases, the water never breaks and the baby is born in a state called "en caul" surrounded by the unruptured amniotic sac! This possibility proves that you can absolutely be in labor even if your water hasn't broken.

With a slow leak of amniotic fluid, sometimes women can't tell if their water has broken. "Is this pee or amniotic fluid?" is a question I'm often asked. If you're truly peeing on yourself, you'll be able to consciously stop the stream of liquid from flowing. If you're leaking amniotic fluid, on the other hand, you won't be able to consciously stop the flow. Because the flow of amniotic fluid cannot be stopped, I highly recommend wearing maxi pads or disposable adult underwear until it's time to start pushing.

If you've tested positive for Group B Strep during this pregnancy, let your midwife or doctor know when your water breaks. Your medical professional will likely advise you to get started on antibiotics so that the infection isn't passed along to the baby during delivery.

When your water breaks, the liquid should be clear or pale yellow, and it may have a slightly sweet smell. If you notice a substance that looks black or greenish, that's a sign that your baby has recently pooped, or passed meconium. Sometimes the baby can inhale or even swallow their meconium during labor which could potentially lead to complications. While it's not a cause for emergency, I recommend calling your midwife or doctor right away. Your midwife or doctor may want you to come in so that they can monitor you and the baby for signs of distress.

Braxton Hicks Contractions vs. Labor Contractions

Braxton Hicks contractions are often known as "practice contractions." This sporadic tightening and releasing of the abdomen seems to be the uterus' way of preparing for labor. Braxton Hicks contractions don't arrive at regular intervals, don't increase in intensity nor do they get closer together in frequency. They don't cause the cervix to dilate.

Labor contractions, on the other hand, start and stop at regular intervals. They get closer together over time and they increase in intensity as labor progresses. Eventually, labor contractions will reach a point where it will become difficult to do anything other than be present with the sensations.

Labor Stages

As you start getting ready for birth, it's also important to learn the Labor Stages. There are three stages of labor: Stage 1 is called Labor, Stage 2 is called Pushing and Birth and Stage 3 is called Delivery of the Placenta. Let's dig deeper into each stage to learn more.

Stage 1: Labor

Stage 1 of labor is called Labor, and this is the stage where the cervix dilates from zero to 10 cm. This stage is divided into two phases: Early Labor and Active Labor.

Early Labor

Early Labor is when the cervix dilates from 0 to 6 cm. Sometimes people don't realize they're in Early Labor because contractions haven't started yet. The amount of cervical dilation is determined by a cervical exam, an assessment where a medical professional (midwife, doctor or nurse), inserts their fingers into the vagina to measure how wide the cervical opening is. Cervical exams are optional and should only be performed with your consent. It's also a procedure that should be used infrequently in order to reduce the risk of infection.

For those who are intending to deliver at a hospital AND they are having a healthy pregnancy without any complications, I recommend laboring at home for as long as possible. Laboring at home during the Early Labor phase allows you to progress without the pressure of being observed and adhering to someone else's schedule. Doctors and nurses use a medical approach to birth that prioritizes hospital protocol. While these regulations can help improve efficiency, their impersonal rigidity can often lead the laboring mom toward hurried decision making and unnecessary stress.

Labor requires deep reserves of energy. And first-time mothers tend to experience longer labors than mothers who have already had children. When you're at home, you're in a familiar space that often feels safe to your body. You can move around and nourish yourself in unrestricted ways. Once you arrive at the hospital, you'll be surrounded by unfamiliar smells, unfamiliar sounds and unfamiliar people going in and out of your room. To the body, the combination of these strange elements during labor can feel like a whole lot of micro-threats. And when the body feels threatened, it's likely to tense up. And when the body tenses up, it's harder for the cervix to relax and dilate.

Active Labor

Active Labor is when the cervix is between 6 and 10 cm dilated. As labor ramps up during this phase, contractions become closer together and more intense. It will be helpful to lean on comfort measures to make the birthing experience more comfortable, especially if you are envisioning your birth to be an unmedicated one.

Here are a few comfort measure options:

Breathing
As the intensity of each contraction increases, some women have a tendency to hold their breath or to hyperventilate. Holding one's breath creates tension in the body as shoulders raise toward the ears, muscles become rigid and the cervix tightens up when it should be opening. I remind my clients to take deep full breaths: inhaling for four counts and exhaling for four counts. Maintaining a steady breathing pattern helps to regulate our emotional state, keeping us in a calmer frame of mind. It also helps ensure that our body and our baby are receiving adequate amounts of oxygen.

Moving
A laboring body wants to be in motion. Frequently changing positions can help the baby move into the optimal position for birth, especially when we take advantage of gravity for additional support in moving the baby down through the birth canal. Your body will give you very clear instructions on how it

wants to move. All you need to do is pay attention. Try walking, bouncing on a birthing ball, dancing, squatting, lunging and even sitting on the toilet. If you have to lie in bed, there are still ways to incorporate movement. Try switching up the side you're lying on every 30 minutes or so, straddle a peanut ball, get on all fours and sway side to side. Moving into different positions on a regular basis can help the body feel more comfortable as the intensity of labor increases. Moving frequently can also help to jumpstart a labor that seems to have stalled out.

Hydrating
The uterus is a muscle, and like other muscles, it works more effectively when it's hydrated. Remember, labor is a marathon, and no one knows how long it'll be until you cross the finish line. Leading up to and during labor, replenish yourself with hydrating drinks (water, coconut water, healthy electrolyte drinks etc.) and hydrating foods (cucumbers, tomatoes, grapes, apples, watermelons etc.) I also encourage my clients to take sips of their hydrating drink in between contractions. Maintaining a steady fluid intake can help you to avoid becoming dehydrated and lethargic during the energy-intensive moments of birth.

Adjusting the temperature

Heating pads, ice packs and warm compresses can provide relief during labor. The change in temperature gives the mind something else to focus on while adjusting the temperature can offer simple ways to alleviate aches, chills or increased body heat.

Using hydrotherapy

Water has a unique way of providing a therapeutic experience in and out of labor. Consider taking a warm shower or a bath as the contractions ramp up in order to help relax the muscles and dampen the intensity of the labor sensations.

Applying counterpressure

Applying steady pressure to targeted areas of the body during a contraction can offer immense relief. Consider asking someone on your birth team to do hip squeezes or apply firm pressure to the lower back.

How to Know It's Go Time

You can use a free contraction timer app to track your contractions. When your contractions are 5 minutes apart, lasting for about 1 minute each and this pattern has been repeated for at least an hour, doulas say that you've met the 5-1-1 Guideline.

Oftentimes, the 5-1-1 Guideline is a marker of being close to 6 cm dilated (though this is not always this case.) When you reach this Guideline, it's often a good time to start heading to the birth center or the hospital. Listen to your body, and trust yourself. If you feel like it's time to go, go.

Transition

As the body prepares to move from Stage 1 to Stage 2 of labor, there is often a brief interim period called Transition. When the cervix approaches 10 cm in dilation and the baby descends lower and lower into the birth canal, there is a major hormonal shift that can influence certain bodily functions. You may begin shivering uncontrollably (even though you're not cold), throwing up or running to the toilet with diarrhea. Birth is a very unique phenomenon, so while some women experience these transition effects, some others don't.

Stage 2: Pushing and Birth

Once the cervix is 10 cm dilated and 100% effaced (fully thinned out), the baby now has enough room to physically fit through the birth canal. Soon, it will be time to push your baby into this world. While this stage can be very intense, it is still possible to enjoy this phase of labor. Some women have had orgasmic and/or euphoric experiences as the baby starts to emerge.

Stage 2 of labor can look very different depending on where you end up giving birth. If you are birthing at a hospital, the nurses will usually encourage you to lay down on the bed once you've reached 10 cm. When you reach this milestone, the nurse will call your doctor to notify them of the baby's imminent arrival. This is when the birthing room begins to get a little crowded, especially if you're delivering at a teaching hospital and have given permission for medical students to attend your birth (remember that it is your right to decline the presence of medical students if you prefer). The doctor and mother/baby nurses will begin to flood the room with their tools and equipment just in time to watch your baby be born. If you're birthing at the birth center or at home, you won't be bombarded with the presence of multiple unfamiliar medical professionals.

Many of my clients have been first time moms and moms who haven't birthed vaginally before, and they have been very curious about how to push and what it's going to feel like. This urge to push feels very similar to the urge to poop. Some women are actually very concerned that they're going to poop while they're pushing. In all honesty, you might. Try not to feel ashamed or embarrassed; this occurrence is completely normal. Midwives, doctors and nurses are all used to seeing all sorts of bodily fluids, and if you do happen to poop while pushing, a nurse will quickly clean it up before you even have time to notice what happened.

If you're birthing at a hospital, the nurses will instruct you to take a deep breath, tuck your chin and pull your thighs towards your chest as you push for 10 seconds at a time. At this stage, most contractions last long enough for you to be able to take another deep breath after the first 10-second pushing interval and then push again for another 10 seconds as the contraction wanes. Pushing with the contractions helps to amplify the effort going into bringing baby earthside.

If you're birthing at a birth center or at home, you will have much more freedom as to where you push and birth your baby. The shower, tub, bed, floor etc. are all fair game. Midwives encourage you to listen to your own body in order to determine when to push and for how long.

Sometimes, my clients begin to feel very overwhelmed with the amount of downward pressure they feel from the baby descending into the birth canal, and this hyper-sensational experience can lead them to start hyperventilating. As a doula, I find myself reminding my clients to inhale fully and exhale fully, letting their shoulders drop away from their ears to help release tension and reset the breathing pattern to one that is more stable and supportive. Making sounds can also be a helpful tool during the pushing stage. I coach my clients to moan deeply as a way to focus their pushing energy towards their vagina.

In between contractions, do your best to rest and sip on your nourishing beverage of choice. This mini-break will allow you to regain some strength in preparation for the next round of pushing. If you're birthing when the baby's head begins to crown as it reaches the opening of the vagina, many women experience what's known as the "ring of fire." A burning sensation can appear as the vaginal tissue stretches to accommodate the size of the baby's head. It can feel like you want to hurry up and push as hard as you can so that you can get beyond this uncomfortable sensation as fast as you can. However, as odd as it may seem, it's actually important to slow down during this moment. Allowing the vaginal tissue time to stretch can help prevent tearing. And as the next contraction arises, you can begin pushing again as the baby's head is born. I like to remind my clients that birthing the head is the hardest part simply because it is the biggest part of the baby. Once the head is born, the baby's body can usually slide out within the next contraction or two.

If you're birthing at a hospital, you can request Immediate Skin to Skin so that the baby is quickly placed on your body instead of being whisked away by the baby nurses to be cleaned and poked and prodded. Immediate Skin to Skin helps the baby to better regulate body temperature plus it helps stimulate milk production and bonding. You can also request Delayed Cord Clamping, where the umbilical cord is not cut until it stops pulsing. While the umbilical cord is still pulsing, it is still capable of delivering vital nutrients to the newborn and leaving it attached during this final transfer can help to increase the baby's iron stores. These are often standard practices amongst birth centers and home births.

Stage 3: Delivering the Placenta

Birth isn't complete until the placenta has been born. The placenta is a temporary organ that your body grows to nourish your baby while you're pregnant. So, once your baby is born, the placenta no longer has a purpose to serve. If you're giving birth in a hospital, the placenta is usually delivered within a few minutes. The doctor will usually tug lightly on the umbilical cord to encourage the placenta to descend along with the uterine contractions. If you're giving birth at a birth center or at home, the midwives are more likely to let the placenta be born at its natural pace, which is usually within the first hour after birth. Many of my clients are curious about what it will feel like to birth the placenta. I find that it has a Jello-like texture, and it tends to slide out without much fuss because the cervix is still fully dilated and effaced. Contractions will continue until the placenta has been delivered, and you might even experience contractions as you breastfeed your baby. These after-birth contractions may last for a few days as they work to help shrink your uterus. By six weeks postpartum, the uterus will have returned to its usual size which is about the size of a fist!

After you deliver the placenta, you are officially considered to be "postpartum." The placenta will, then, be inspected to make sure that it is intact; if chunks of placenta are left in the body, they can cause an infection. Once the placenta has been delivered, you can choose to let the hospital "dispose" of it (it's unclear what exactly happens to your placenta after the nurses take it from you) or you can choose to keep it. There are trained placenta encapsulation practitioners who can dehydrate the placenta and pour the powder into ingestible pills. Some women say that their mental and emotional health greatly improved after taking their own placenta pills. Other people are interested in keeping the placenta for postpartum rituals or perhaps even planting it in the family garden. Keep in mind that if you would like to keep your placenta, and you're birthing at a hospital or a birthing center, you'll need to bring a disposable cooler with you in order to transport your placenta.

Chapter 3: Train Your Mind for Birth

As I was preparing to welcome my third baby in 2024, I created a workshop for the organization I co-founded, Maternal Resource Oasis, all about how to Train Your Mind for Birth. We all know that birth is a physical event, but many people don't realize just how important it is to prepare for birth mentally as well. Our thoughts play a significant role in the way we behave during birth. This concept is so important, that I've adapted the workshop into the following section of this book. So, I highly recommend that you take some time to train your mind for birth while you're still pregnant so that you can allow the following material to sink in before you're in the throes of labor.

Improve Your Self Esteem

After hearing many clients express such doubt about their ability to give birth, it has become clear to me that they generally don't believe they're capable of accomplishing their life goals. It's important to understand how you think about yourself and what you're capable of because what you *believe* is possible often turns into what *is* possible for yourself. I really appreciated reading the book *The Six Pillars of Self-Esteem* by Nathanial Branden, and I highly recommend reading it yourself. It helped me to improve my self-esteem by learning how to experience myself as a person who is competent enough to cope with life challenges and as a person worthy of happiness.

Watch Your Words

Most of my clients have been interested in having a vaginal unmedicated birth while also feeling deeply doubtful about their ability to do so. "I think I want to have a vaginal unmedicated birth, but I also don't think I can do it," is a common statement I hear. The way that we speak about ourselves impacts how we show up in the world. Sowing seeds of self-doubt can work against yourself because it subtly convinces yourself that you're not going to be able to do what you intend. This form of doublespeak can lend itself to an internal conflict that is difficult to overcome. Instead, use your words to empower yourself. Statements like "I'm interested in having a vaginal unmedicated birth, but I'm unsure of how to go about it. Even still, I'm going to learn what I can in order to prepare for this journey" allow you to acknowledge your uncertainty while still making room for you to learn as you go.

Select Your Affirmations

During pregnancy, it's helpful to pick out encouraging words or phrases that you can return to as labor progresses. You can write them on sticky notes to leave in places you frequent, and you can also ask the people around you to reflect your affirmations back to you.

Here are some examples that I have used personally:

- My body was made to do this.
- This is all temporary. This will all be over by lunchtime (or whatever time frame makes sense for you.)
- So many women have crossed this threshold before, and they're waiting to welcome me, too.

Weed Out the Negativity

As I was preparing for my third birth, I started to notice a sense of dread sprouting up in my mind. For a couple of weeks, I would let those seeds begin to take root until I realized I needed to weed them out. I couldn't continue to prepare for this birth alongside feelings of dread. I encourage you to take stock of the thoughts that are coming up in your mind. Are you replaying negative ideas in your mind? Are you finding that these thoughts are making you anxious or fearful or sad? Reflect on where these feelings might be coming from. When you address any concerns that arise, you allow the negativity to fade away.

Creating Your Birth Vision

While the term "Birth Plan" has become ultra-popular in recent years, I personally avoid using it. Now, hear me out: I absolutely recognize the importance of listing out the elements that one hopes to include or avoid during the birthing experience. I also see the value in sharing this summary with the people on your birth team. Our words have the power to shape how we perceive ourselves, our reality and the world around us. However, the word "plan" primes the mind to think that you can dictate exactly how a birth unfolds just by stating your preferences. In all honesty, birth is a mysterious event that can unfold in mysterious ways. It cannot be *planned.*

Instead, I help my clients describe their "Birth Vision." By using the word "vision,"we can also practice releasing ourselves from the expectation that we can control how birth unfolds. The Birth Vision is a collection of elements that you envision being present during your birthing experience. Infuse your Birth Vision with sensory details that help you to better envision yourself feeling safe and supported in labor while having a positive, enjoyable experience. You can download a free Birth Vision template at younghonestmother.com.

The following questions will help you clarify your Birth Vision:

1. **What kind of birthing experience do you envision?**

I encourage my clients to think deeply about why they would like to have this experience. Is it just something you heard about? What is the connection there for you? Have you done your research to better understand which experience is best for you? Getting clear about your "why" can help you stay motivated to move in this direction even if challenges arise.

Types of Birthing Experiences:
- Vaginal, unmedicated
- Vaginal, medicated (includes receiving medication to induce labor and/or minimize discomfort)
- Scheduled c-section
- Undecided

2. Where do you envision yourself giving birth?

Where you give birth plays a big part in how you give birth. In the United States of America, there are three main birthing locations: home, birth centers and the hospital. Since each birthing location is led by different types of medical professionals, each birthing location also has a very distinct Model of Care, or approach of caring, for laboring women. So, it's very important to choose a birthing location that is best suited to the kind of birth experience you envision yourself having. Let's explore the basics of each birthing location:

Home Birth

A planned birth that takes place wherever you live. Giving birth at home offers families the utmost autonomy to experience along with an unhurried and personalized birthing experience. Up until the mid-1900's, women in the USA mainly gave birth in the comfort of their own homes with the help of the local midwife.

Best Suited for:
- Vaginal, unmedicated births for women having low-risk pregnancies.
- Families interested in out-of-hospital births who want to experience the utmost autonomy and comfort of birthing in a familiar environment.

Attended By:
- Certified Professional Midwives (CPMs)
  - Licensed medical providers trained to offer holistic, comprehensive care throughout pregnancy, birth and postpartum in a way that respects the woman's desires and preferences.
- Certified Nurse Midwives (CNMs)
  - Licensed medical providers who trained as nurses first and then graduated from a midwifery program.

Model of Care:
Midwives Model of Care ©, an approach based on the fact that pregnancy and birth are both normal life processes. The Midwives Model of Care © has

been proven to reduce the incidence of birth injury, trauma and c-section, and it prioritizes:

- monitoring the physical, psychological, and social well-being of the mother throughout the childbearing cycle.
- providing the mother with individualized education, counseling, prenatal care, continuous hands-on assistance during labor and delivery and postpartum support.
- minimizing technological interventions.
- identifying and referring women who require obstetrical attention.

Birth Center Birth

A non-hospital birthing location designed to resemble a home-like setting with features that often include a spacious bed, tub and/or shower. Birth Centers are often found near local hospitals to allow for quick hospital transfers if necessary.

Best Suited For:
- vaginal, unmedicated births for women having low-risk pregnancies

- families interested in an out-of-hospital birth who aren't interested in birthing at home

Attended By:
- Certified Professional Midwives (CPMs)
- Certified Nurse Midwives (CNMs)

Model of Care: Midwives Model of Care ©

Hospital Birth

A birthing location designed to offer access to advanced medical care and a range of interventions.

Best Suited For:
- vaginal, medicated births
- high-risk pregnancies
- c-sections
- families who feel safer in hospital settings

Attended By:
- OB/GYNs
    - Doctors who specialize in obstetrics and gynecology, a medicalized approach to prenatal, birth and postpartum treatment. OB/GYNs are also trained in how to perform surgeries (i.e. c-sections)
- Certified Nurse Midwives (CNMs)

- Labor and delivery nurses
  - Registered nurses who work closely with OB/GYNs and/or CNMs to assist in providing comprehensive care and monitoring during birth

Model of Care: Medical Model of Care, a standardized approach to labor and delivery that is structured around hospital-specific protocol. So, when someone chooses to give birth at a hospital, the hospital staff expects that person to submit to those protocols. The Medical Model of Care categorizes birth as "a pathological process requiring intensive monitoring and the use of medical intervention" (Ferrer et al. 2016). The psychological, spiritual, cultural and emotional aspects of bringing new life into the world are more easily forgotten or ignored within this model.

Curating a Respectful Birth Team

As you create your Birth Vision, I highly recommend that you ask around for recommendations on providers who are respectful of birth wishes, cultural background and birth circumstances (VBAC, unmedicated, twins, breech etc.). Remember: you are the one hiring the medical provider. If you don't like the way they provide care, you can choose to seek out care from a different provider. Medical providers often stop accepting new patients into their practice once a woman is around 30-33 weeks pregnant. So, if you *are* interested in finding a doctor or midwife who is a better fit for your Birth Vision, make sure you do your due diligence early on in your pregnancy.

I've had many clients that I've connected with later in their pregnancies who have told me their doctor had never once asked them about what they envisioned for their birth. In light of that, I recommend that you set aside time during an upcoming prenatal visit to share your Birth Vision with your doctor and/or midwife. If you have a doula, it's a great idea to invite them to join this appointment as well. Speak to your birth team about why the birth that you envision resonates with you. Being in conversation about your preferences before the big day helps everyone on your birth team to be on the same page (literally) about how to best support you.

Cost is usually the biggest factor that my clients have to consider in terms of selecting the birthing location. If you are interested in birthing outside of the hospital but aren't sure if you can afford it, ask your local midwives about sliding scale services, scholarships and/or payment plans.

3. **What are your Three Birth Feels, three words that describe how you want to feel during your birthing experience?**

When you identify how you would like to feel during birth, you can move through labor with more intention, carefully selecting elements that contribute to your emotional wellbeing. A list of ideas to spark your imagination is included in the Birth Vision template that you can download at younghonestmother.com.

4. **Who do you envision being present in the birthing room?**

Be mindful of the energy in your space. Birthing is a very vulnerable experience, and other people's attitudes and perspectives on birth can easily influence the atmosphere. I recommend only inviting people who you feel safe around and supported by.

5. **What comfort measures do you envision using?**

Comfort measures are methods that you can use to feel more comfortable during labor. It's helpful to pick a few out to include in your Birth Vision so that you can practice embodied visualizations leading up to your birthing experience.

6. **Are there any cultural, religious or spiritual practices you envision including during your birth?**

During the spiritual experience of bringing new life into the world, prayer can be especially rejuvenating. Some of my clients choose a few sacred scriptures to repeat in silent prayer or out loud. Connecting with the divine can alleviate mental and emotional distress during the vulnerable moments of giving birth. Perhaps you would prefer to be tended to by an all-female staff during your labor due to your faith. Make note of any specific cultural, religious or spiritual practices. Your preferences matter.

7. **What sensory elements do you envision including in your birthing experience? What sensory elements would you like to exclude from your birthing experience?**

You can create an enjoyable birthing environment that helps you to feel safe by involving your senses during birth. When the body feels safe, it can relax and open. Start by considering where in your space you feel most comfortable. What room are you most drawn to when you feel stressed and you want to relax?

Here are some sensory elements you might consider including in your birthing experience:

Sight

Consider lighting some candles and/or turning off overhead lights in favor of lamps in order to create a warm and inviting cozy ambiance. You could even consider writing out your affirmations and taping them to the walls in various rooms of your home so that you can see constant reminders of encouraging words.

Smell

Candles, incense and essential oils can all contribute to an uplifting birthing environment. If you are birthing at a hospital, consider bringing a diffuser or a roller ball filled with your favorite essential oils so that you can tap into the benefits of aromatherapy even when you're away from home. If you're preparing for a home birth, you have the opportunity to create different scent experiences from room to room.

Sound

You can put together a playlist of your favorite songs to inspire you to dance, sing and enjoy yourself while you're moving through contractions. Meditative songs, ASMR videos, a crackling fire and drum beats can even help induce trance-like states which can be extremely helpful during labor as well.

Touch

We are often soothed by touching soft things. Is there anything soft you could envision being present during your labor?

Taste

Is there a meal or a treat you've really had a taste for during your pregnancy? Consider having it on hand to nibble on during labor (if you happen to feel like eating) or right after your baby is born so that you have a special dining experience to look forward to.

When you're creating a space with pleasurable sensory elements in your birth experience, you're also helping to create a felt sense of safety in your body. Again, when you're feeling fearful and panicked, the body tenses up, making it harder for the cervix to open. On the flip side, when you create an environment that has the sensory elements that you enjoy, it helps you to relax and to dilate, which is exactly what needs to happen for you to be able to birth your baby. Stacking together simple and inexpensive sensory elements such as the ones I shared above is a tactic that anyone can use as a way to enhance their birthing experience.

Practice Embodied Visualization

While you wait for your baby to be born, it's common to find yourself getting lost in daydreams. So, why not use that time as a training ground for envisioning what labor and birth will feel and look like? See yourself staying the course and overcoming challenges. See yourself being pushed to what feels like your limit, and then see yourself going beyond that as you surrender to what your birthing experience holds. Include joy in your daydreams. See yourself holding your baby in your arms as you experience the true embodiment of joy.

If there are things that you definitely *don't* want people to say because you know that it would take you out of the moment or have you feeling panicked or fearful for some reason. You can share those with the people that you would like to be in the birth room so that they know as well. For example, when I was in labor, I really did not want anyone telling me that I looked beautiful during labor because I didn't want my mind to be distracted by how I looked.

When you are getting ready for birth, I recommend that you regularly share your Birth Vision with the supportive people in your life like your midwife and/or doctor, your doula and your closest loved one(s). Visualizing together as a collective will allow your birth team to reinforce and reflect back to you the vision that you're holding.

Chapter 5: Exploring Alternative Birth Scenarios

I notice that my clients hold a subtle yet strong belief that if they prepare for the birth they want AND they hire a doula, then their birthing experience will unfold exactly the way they envision it. In all honesty, that's not the way it works. At the end of the day, there are always unseen variables that can potentially redirect your course of action. The true purpose of preparation is to ready yourself for whatever situation you may find yourself in.

Simply put: birth can unfold in a variety of different ways for a variety of different reasons. There are medical reasons that can suddenly emerge that require a change in how birth unfolds. Remember that the baby is also part of the birth! Sometimes, changes need to be made based on how the baby is responding to labor.

Some people think that acknowledging the un-ideal will make it more likely to happen that way. I don't agree. In fact, when you ignore various birth possibilities, you leave yourself vulnerable to having to make important decisions on the fly without much education. Here's how I see it: when you expand your Birth Vision to include various birth possibilities, you are preparing yourself to approach potential decisions with informed consent.

Check In with Your Emotions

Birth is a sacred event that taps into our emotional core. Part of what can make expanding the Birth Vision so challenging is the meaning we often attach to the way birth unfolds. We come face to face with our own power to bring forth life at the same time that we brush up against just how little control we have over how that very life is brought forth. This paradox can feel unsettling because we are used to the idea of being able to control our own bodies, and we often have minimal practice with the art of surrendering.

It's not a failure for birth to take twists and turns in ways that don't align with your Birth Vision.

However, I do think it's important to recognize the emotional undertone beneath various birth possibilities. Making space to meet our own feelings with lovingkindness helps us to remain clear and open. This level of compassionate clarity will help to shed light on the real versus imagined implications of each birth unfolding. As a doula, my ultimate goal is to help guide parents toward a state of peaceful preparedness. It's impossible to reach that goal if you're ignoring the fear, confusion, sadness, disappointment etc. that you may be hiding from.

Many people are unfamiliar with exploring their own feelings, and the idea of expanding your Birth Vision might seem overwhelming. So, before we explore alternative birth scenarios in the next section, identify a Soothing Resource that you can turn to if you start feeling uncomfortable with the visualization prompts. Examples: a warm and cozy robe, a hot mug of tea, a neck massager, a rollerball filled with your favorite essential oils etc. As we continue, you may notice that a certain birth unfolding brings about particular sensations or emotional responses. Rest there awhile. Revisit your Soothing Resource, and return to this book once the emotional intensity has turned down. Facing your emotions in small doses can make the reflective experience more tolerable. So, move through the next section little by little, if that feels right for you.

In some cases, medical circumstances can suddenly emerge that will require a change to the Birth Vision. Let's spend some time exploring various birth scenarios.

Use Your BRAIN

When I'm helping my clients to evaluate medical decisions during labor, especially when birth seems to be unfolding in a way that my clients didn't envision, I encourage them to use the BRAIN acronym. Unless it's a true medical emergency, remember that it's ok to slow down and think about what decision you want to make. Posing these questions to your medical provider will help you better understand their medical advice, and possibly help you avoid feeling like you rushed your decision making.

B- What are the Benefits of moving in this direction?
R- What are the Risks of moving in this direction?
A- What are the Alternatives to moving in this direction?
I- What is my Intuition telling me?
N- What if I do Nothing for now?

If you find yourself needing to veer away from your ideal Birth Vision, you can still feel calm and confident about how to move forward once you've taken the time to understand various birth scenarios.

So, in this section, we'll:
- note the different birth scenarios.
- highlight common medical reasons behind different birth scenarios.
- uncover your emotional responses to various birth scenarios.

Alternative Birth Scenarios
1. Induction

When labor is not progressing, a medical provider may advise that certain techniques be used in order to stimulate the uterus to contract. This process is called an induction.

Common Medical Reasons for Inductions:
- Approaching 42 weeks pregnant
- Water broke over 24 hours ago, and labor is not progressing with steady contractions/ dilation
- Gestational diabetes (especially if managed with insulin)

Induction Methods that Do NOT Involve Medication:

- *Nipple Stimulation*
    - Stimulating the nipples orally or with a breast pump helps the body produce oxytocin, a hormone that stimulates labor contractions.

- *Membrane Sweep*
    - A procedure where a medical professional uses their gloved finger to sweep between the area where the amniotic sac attaches to the uterus. When the amniotic membranes are separated, the body can start to release prostaglandins, chemicals that help to soften, thin and dilate the cervix. Results can take hours or even days.
- *Foley Bulb*
    - A balloon-tipped catheter that is inserted into the cervix. As the balloon inflates with saline solution, the balloon puts pressure on the cervix and encourages it to dilate. The catheter falls out when the cervix is around 3-5 cm dilated. Results can take hours.
- *Artificial Rupture of Membranes (AROM)*

- A procedure where a medical professional intentionally ruptures the amniotic sac or "breaks the water" in order to strengthen labor contractions and encourage the cervix to dilate. This method is usually reserved for when other methods have not been effective because rupturing the baby's amniotic sac can increase the risk of infection.

Induction Methods that DO Involve Medication: These methods introduce synthetic hormones to jumpstart labor, and these artificial elements can cause labor contractions to be much more intense than natural labor contractions. Always talk to your medical provider about the risks and benefits of medications and your unique medical history.

- *Misoprostol (Cytotec)*
  - A synthetic prostaglandin that can be given orally or vaginally to soften the cervix and stimulate the uterus. This drug was originally created to treat stomach ulcers and has not been approved by the FDA to be used in labor inductions. Results can take hours.
  - NOTE: At the time of this publishing in 2025, the official label for Cytotec reads: ADMINISTRATION TO WOMEN WHO

ARE PREGNANT CAN CAUSE ABORTION, PREMATURE BIRTH, OR BIRTH DEFECTS. UTERINE RUPTURE HAS BEEN REPORTED WHEN CYTOTEC WAS ADMINISTERED IN PREGNANT WOMEN TO INDUCE LABOR OR TO INDUCE ABORTION.

- *Cervidil*
  - A device that is inserted into the vagina containing time-released medication that may help soften and dilate the cervix. This device has been FDA approved for cervical ripening. Results can take hours.
- *Pitocin*
  - A medication derived from the hormone oxytocin synthetic. This medication is given through an IV in graduated doses in order to hyperstimulate the uterus to contract. Results can take hours or days.

Check In with Your Emotions

Let's pause here for a few deep breaths. Remember to reach for your Soothing Resource before you ask yourself the following questions:

- What's your relationship to medication?
- Have you experienced sexual and/or physical trauma? If so, have you shared this with your

medical provider so that they know to take internal exams slowly?

- What sensations do you notice in your body when you consider this particular birth scenario? Where in your body do you notice them?
- What's behind the feelings that arise when you consider this birth scenario?
- If your experience were to veer in the direction of induction, how could you still connect to your Three Birth Feels?

2. Comfort Management Medication

There are various medicines to help improve a woman's comfort level during labor by either minimizing or numbing the pain associated with giving birth.

Common Medical Reasons for Comfort Management Medication:

- Long labor without much rest
- Pain becomes unbearable
- Mom has a hard time breathing and regulating her heart rate

Types of Comfort Management Medications:

- *Nitrous Oxide (Laughing Gas)*

- A mixture of nitrous oxide and oxygen that can be inhaled via a mask. It provides mild relief during labor by helping to take the edge off of painful sensations while still allowing the woman to move around during labor.
- *IV Pain Medicine*
  - An opioid that is administered via an IV that can provide quick pain relief and a calming effect during labor. Because the opioid enters the bloodstream and passes through the placenta, it can also have an effect on the baby's alertness, breathing and heart rate. In order to avoid health complications for the baby post-birth, this option is typically only given to a woman during the earlier stages of labor.
- *Epidural*
  - A type of anesthesia injected into the epidural region of the spine. This medication blocks pain signals from traveling to the brain and creates a sensation of numbness from the waist down. While a woman can still be aware of contractions, she will no longer be able to walk around the room, and

moving into different labor positions in the bed will require assistance.

Check In with Your Emotions

Let's pause here for a few deep breaths. Remember to reach for your Soothing Resource before you ask yourself the following questions:

- What sensations do you notice in your body when you consider this particular birth scenario? Where in your body do you notice them?
- What's behind the feelings that arise when you consider this birth scenario?
- If your experience were to veer in the direction of comfort management medication, how could you still connect to your Three Birth Feels?

3. Unplanned C-Section

A surgical birth that is recommended for a non-emergency situation. Remember that you can ask for time to process the information and prepare yourself for surgery during a quiet moment with loved ones. A support person is usually allowed in the operating room.

Common Medical Reasons for an Unplanned C-section:

- Pushing for hours and baby has not descended (often because baby is malpositioned)
- Baby is in the breech position (not head down)
- Baby's heart rate is consistently dropping after contractions
- Mom and/or baby are showing signs of infection

Consider a Gentle C-Section:

Scheduled c-sections, and often even unplanned c-sections, can take on a gentle approach that allows for:

- a clear drape separating the mother's face from the operation so that she can see her baby being born.
- calming music.
- delayed cord clamping.
- a loved one to have immediate skin to skin with the baby.

Check In with Your Emotions

Let's pause here for a few deep breaths. Remember to reach for your Soothing Resource before you ask yourself the following questions:

- What is your relationship to surgery?

- What sensations do you notice in your body when you consider this particular birth scenario? Where in your body do you notice them?
- What's behind the feelings that arise when you consider this birth scenario?
- If your experience were to veer in the direction of an unplanned c-section, how could you still connect to your Three Birth Feels?

4. Emergency C-Section

When an emergency health concern presents itself, an emergency c-section will be recommended. During an emergency c-section, the mother will most often be put under general anesthesia, which means she will be unconscious during the birth of the baby. Support people are usually not allowed in the operating room during emergency c-sections.

Common Medical Reasons for Emergency C-sections
- Baby's heart rate consistently and drastically drops low after contractions
- Baby and/or mother are in acute distress

Check In with Your Emotions

Let's pause here for a few deep breaths. Remember to reach for your Soothing Resource before you ask yourself the following questions:

- What sensations do you notice in your body when you consider this particular birth scenario? Where in your body do you notice them?
- What's behind the feelings that arise when you consider this birth scenario?
- If your experience were to veer in the direction of an emergency c-section, how could you still connect to your Three Birth Feels?

Conclusion

As you prepare for birth, remember to be mindful about what you consume. I'm not just talking about nutrition here, although that is definitely important. The shows and movies that we watch, the books that we read and the conversations that we listen to are capable of influencing how we think and feel about birth.

These days, there are countless podcasts and YouTube videos dedicated to sharing positive birth stories. That means that it is easier than ever to curate the kind of input you receive. In an effort to expand your vision of birth, I recommend consuming birth stories from women who had birthing experiences that veered away from their ideal and STILL consider their birthing experience to have been a positive one. Surrounding yourself with a diverse set of birth stories will help you to see that there is more than one way to experience birth as positive. You may even walk away with new ideas that you can incorporate into your own Birth Vision.

As a doula, I realized that most of my clients felt completely unsure of how to go about getting ready for birth. Many of my clients thought that their doctors would spend more time sharing lessons in childbirth education. In reality, after the doctor examines physical health metrics, there is rarely any time to address anything else during their quick 15-minute prenatal appointment.

After reading this book, you've learned how to:
- classify the stages of labor in order to better visualize what your body could experience while bringing new life into the world.
- train your mind for birth in order to improve mental endurance.
- create your own Birth Vision in order to gain clarity about your birthing preferences.
- explore alternative birth scenarios in order to be prepared with vital insights in case your birthing experience isn't quite what you envisioned.

There is so much more to share about pregnancy, birth and postpartum, but this book is intentionally short in the hopes of not contributing to the sense of overwhelm many parents feel as they're preparing to welcome a new baby into the family. I encourage you to share what you discovered while reading this book with the rest of your birth team. And may you feel at ease and empowered to make informed decisions and advocate for respectful care while you're getting ready for birth.

Glossary

Artificial Rupture of Membranes (AROM)
A procedure where a medical professional intentionally ruptures the amniotic sac or "breaks the water" in order to strengthen labor contractions and encourage the cervix to dilate. This method is usually reserved for when other methods have not been effective because rupturing the baby's amniotic sac can increase the risk of infection.

Birth Center
A non-hospital birthing location designed to resemble a home-like setting with features that often include a spacious bed, tub and/or shower. Birth Centers are led by midwives and are often found near local hospitals to allow for quick hospital transfers if necessary.

Birth Team

The team of people you assemble to support you during birth e.g. midwife, doctor, doula, best friend, loved ones.

Birth Vision

A collection of elements that you envision being present during your birthing experience.

Braxton Hicks Contractions

The painless rhythmic tightening and release of the uterus in preparation for labor.

BRAIN

An acronym to help you navigate decision making during labor:

B- What are the **B**enefits of moving in this direction?
R- What are the **R**isks of moving in this direction?
A- What are the **A**lternatives to moving in this direction?
I- What is my **I**ntuition telling me?
N- What if I do **N**othing for now?

Cervix

The lower part of the uterus that connects to the vagina which widens in order for a baby to be born.

Collective Visualization

Regularly sharing your Birth Vision with the supportive people in your life like your midwife and/or doctor, your doula and your closest loved one(s). Visualizing together as a collective will allow your birth team to reinforce and reflect back to you the vision that you're holding.

Comfort Measures

Methods that you can use to feel more comfortable during labor.

Delayed Cord Clamping

When the umbilical cord is not cut until it stops pulsing after the baby is born.

Dilation

The process of the cervix opening from 0 to 10 cm during labor.

Doula

A trained professional who helps families navigate preconception, pregnancy, birth and postpartum with childbirth education and postpartum support.

Effacement

The process of the cervix thinning from 0-100% during labor.

Foley Bulb
A balloon-tipped catheter that is inserted into the cervix. As the balloon inflates with saline solution, the balloon puts pressure on the cervix and encourages it to dilate. The catheter falls out when the cervix is around 3-5 cm dilated. Results can take hours.

Immediate Skin to Skin
When the newborn baby is placed directly onto the skin of the mother or another loved one immediately after birth.

Induction
The process of using certain techniques to stimulate the uterus to contract in order to initiate and/or accelerate labor.

Interventions
Non-medical or medical procedures that are used to help with the birthing process.

Membrane Sweep
A procedure where a medical professional uses their gloved finger to sweep between the area where the amniotic sac attaches to the uterus. When the amniotic membranes are separated, the body can start to release prostaglandins, chemicals that help

to soften, thin and dilate the cervix. Results can take hours or even days.

Midwife
A healthcare professional that specializes in providing care during pre-conception, pregnancy, labor, birth and postpartum. There are two main types of midwives in the USA:

- **Certified Professional Midwives (CPMs)**
  - Licensed medical providers trained to offer holistic, comprehensive care throughout pregnancy, birth and postpartum in a way that respects the woman's desires and preferences.
- **Certified Nurse Midwives (CNMs)**
  - Licensed medical providers who trained as nurses first and then graduated from a midwifery program.

Model of Care
A distinct approach of caring for laboring women that varies based on birthing location and the medical professionals that attend births there.

The Midwives Model of Care© is an approach based on the fact that pregnancy and birth are both normal life processes. The Midwives Model of

Care© has been proven to reduce the incidence of birth injury, trauma and c-section, and it prioritizes:

- monitoring the physical, psychological, and social well-being of the mother throughout the childbearing cycle.
- providing the mother with individualized education, counseling, prenatal care, continuous hands-on assistance during labor and delivery and postpartum support.
- minimizing technological interventions.
- identifying and referring women who require obstetrical attention.

The Medical Model of Care is a standardized approach to labor and delivery that is structured around hospital-specific protocol. The Medical Model of Care is practiced by OB/GYNs and categorizes birth as "a pathological process requiring intensive monitoring and the use of medical intervention" (Ferrer et al. 2016). The psychological, spiritual, cultural, emotional and mental aspects of bringing new life into the world are not prioritized within this model.

Mucus Plug

A thick, mucus-like blob that seals off the cervix during pregnancy to keep bacteria from entering the uterus and causing an infection.

OB/GYN

A doctor who specializes in obstetrics and gynecology, a medicalized approach to prenatal, birth and postpartum treatment. An OB/GYN is also trained in how to perform surgeries (i.e. c-sections).

Placenta

A temporary organ that your body grows to nourish the baby during pregnancy.

Soothing Resource

An object you can turn to if you start feeling uncomfortable with the visualization prompts. e.g. a warm and cozy robe, a hot mug of tea, a neck massager.